Table of Contents

The Inner Game of Weight Loss™

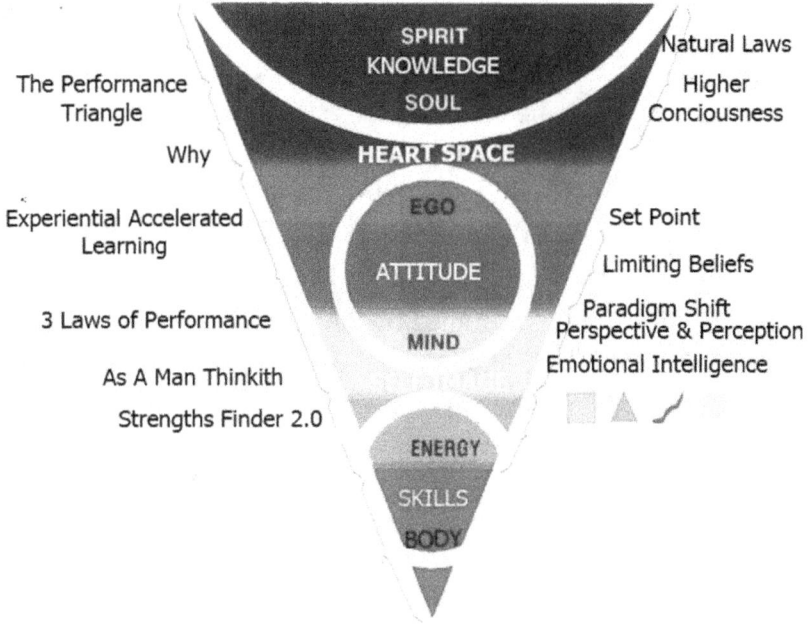

A Note From The Author

Dear Reader,

I acknowledge you for taking the first steps towards an even healthier lifestyle.

Please start here read the following letter to understand the paradigm or setting of *The Inner Game of Weight Loss*™

Let me ask you a question:

If you were doing everything right and then found out it was actually wrong, how soon would you want to know that what you were doing was wrong?

For me I would want to know right now. As you read through this book I invite you to be open to the ideas and research. This book is starting a new conversation, one that I do not know anyone else having.

Research tells us that 70% of people will read 30% of a book. And that most people never get past page 18. Knowing these statistics we are going to put our very best breakthrough ideas in the 1st 30 pages.

Our results will NOT come from learning ABOUT The Inner Game of Weight Loss™ from a book, it will come from you seeing value in it and having an experience with this technology and APPLYING it.

What I Ask of You

Since we are going to reveal big ideas that many schools, businesses, clubs & clients have invested thousands of dollars for I have a few concerns and would like to address them now.

The unfortunate truth is that free advice does NOT always work. Myself and others have invested substantial amounts of time, money, and energy developing his proprietary training system. If you were given this resource at a low or no cost you might make the mistake of not placing a high value on it. What I have found is we often only place high value on the things we pay for, and/or have had to earn.

Because of our commitment to share this resource with as many athletes as possible you may have either paid a ridiculously low investment or you might have been given this book as a gift.

Either way because you are not yet fully invested you might discount this book, its ideas. And that is your choice. It would be a mistake. And you will not truly value the genius of what I am revealing to you. Your breakthrough depends on your ability to follow, value and apply this course and the pages that follow.

Here rather than me tell you, let me show you.

<u>Note:</u> Get ready to challenge your current thinking.

Imagine, for a minute that you were handed a map of "Europe" and it is mislabeled the "United States."

So here we are in the United States with a map that we think is of the United States and in really a map of Europe. Now imagine with this map of Europe we are "trying" to get to New Jersey from Chicago.

With this map as our guide would we ever be able to get from where we are to where we want to go?

With this map as our reference, would WORKING HARDER make any difference in getting us from Chicago to New Jersey?

With this map as our reference would having more FOCUS help us in getting from Chicago to New Jersey.

With this map as our reference, would spending more TIME "trying" to figure out directions make any difference?

Clearly, no. Right?

When our map is inaccurate, it will make no difference how hard we try to find our destination or how positively we think—we will stay stuck.

Learning another take down, working on another turn from top, or an escape from bottom would be like, in this example (*again with the wrong map*) choosing to take a bike rather than walking, or deciding to drive a car rather than taking a bike. You can see how using another vehicle such as a bike or car would only get us lost even faster. Technique is really important and it is not the only variable in our highest potential.

Being motivated is not the answer because we would still be operating from the wrong map. It would just get us lost even faster, have us feeling frustrated.

Being more focused, working harder and longer, being stronger and faster is not always the solution.

One solution is: To stop and ask someone who has been there before to train us and teach us that this is a map of Europe and not a map of the United States."

Hi my name is Brian Daly and for almost two decades, I competed as a top nationally ranked wrestler, each and every year qualifying to compete 3x's at the State Tournament and 4x's at the NCAA National Championships. During the season I beat multiple State Placers, All Americans and even National Champions. I do not share that with you to impress you but to share with you for the following:

For me when it came down to the State Finals & NCAA Championships, each and every time something seemed to happened in to those critical matches, moments and minutes that decide the ones who go on to place and those who go home with nothing. Having this happen 7x's it left me feeling disappointment, frustrated and with a lot of unanswered questions.

See I did what my coaches and I knew. I trained hard and long, I worked on being stronger and faster And it didn't work.

Most coaches are still teaching this old model of work harder and longer, being stronger and faster than your completion, being tough. The truth is that only focusing on the physical side of weightloss is only 33% of the complete package.

With my map I was NEVER going to make it from where I was to where I wanted to go. Fortunately after 17 years wrestling and 5 years searching for answers, we found solutions and packaged them into a complete mentoring program which is now available to you.

As a top-performing grade school, high school, and college athlete, I know what it's like to be in those perceived high pressure critical moments.

The questions that I have asked myself since the end of my college athletic career is what inspired me to develop this program. We are starting a new conversation, one that I do not know anyone else having with wrestlers like you.

There is a better way, we found it and were excited you found this resource.

Warning: You take on all the risk associated with starting to read this program seeing its value and not following through with taking action.

My prediction for you is, if you do not understand and apply this training, you will risk your dream of being a State or National Champion. You will end up working harder than you need to, waste so much valuable time and risk missing out.

My experience has been that often at times we want something to change, and in order for that to happen we need new information, new resources and a new perspective from someone who has or had the results we are looking for.

Fortunately, we've uncovered what it takes to breakthrough to the results you want. And finally – for the first time ever – we are about to reveal it to you.

How to Read This Guide for Maximum Application

The Inner Game of Weight Loss™ Program is organized according to five specific steps. The only way for you to get the full value of this program is to do the following:

1. <u>Print</u> - If you do not have a printed copy of this program. Get one. And for now take a moment, and print this book. I have purposely set it up to allow you enough room to take notes.

2. <u>Quick Overview</u> - It is designed for you to read this over quickly the first time to understand the overall paradigm.

3. <u>Close Reading</u> - Re-read this book a second time as you underline the critical concepts. In the margins, you can also write down any

key ideas that stick out in your mind as a way to reinforce them as well as to have easy access to referring back to them later.

4. <u>Share/Discuss</u> - To take it a step further, share what you've read and what notes you've taken with someone else (a coach, a parent, or another teammate)

5. <u>Reflect</u> - Finally, read for the third time through and self reflect and decide how to apply this book.

When you follow these five steps, you will get the most value from your invested time, energy and money.

The power of the system that I am exposing you to will be revealed as you self-reflect on these ideas. A new paradigm of understanding can only be seen when we go through a process like this.

When we allow our brain to look, compare, make metaphors, test, and observe relationships long enough, *we will often see something that you did not see before.*

So read on…

To Developing The Leader Within,

Brian Daly

The Inner Game of Weight Loss™

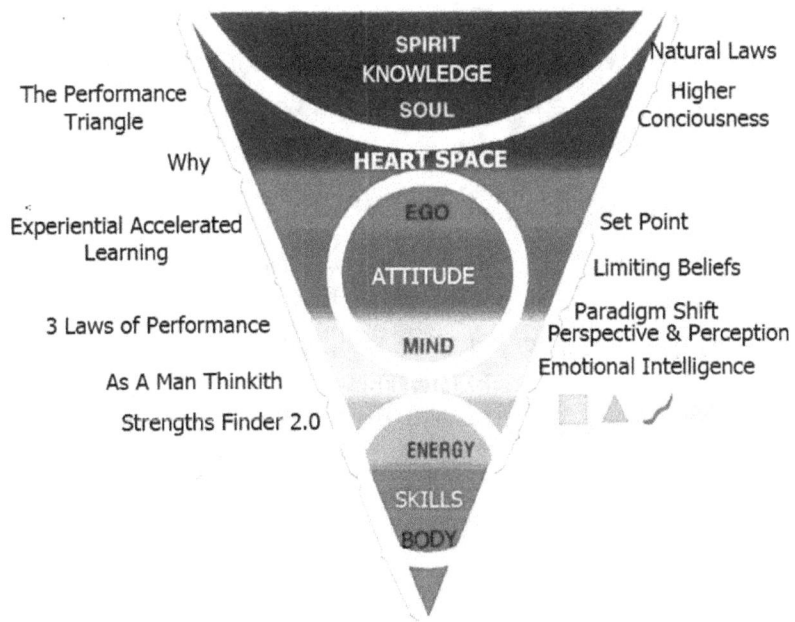

The Inner Game of Weight Loss™ is different from any other camp, training or practice in that it is the 1st Complete & Comprehensive Program.

The Inner Game of Weight Loss is designed to NOT leave you with just more information or knowledge about losing weight. The Inner Game of Weight Loss™ and its technology is strategically designed from an application standpoint and with specific intentions, outcomes and measures.

Brian and his team have invested substantial amounts of time, money, and energy developing his proprietary training system and mentoring program. He will lead you through the process as you discover The Inner Game of Weight Loss™.

If you want to move through the program faster, and/or get an experience of personally working with Brian & his team.

I invite you to request a Free 3 Way 30 Minute Strategy Session. Many times this call looks like a call between you & our leadership team.

To Schedule a time that works for everyone Call 773-574-6600.

Or To Apply to The Inner Game of Weight Loss™ Team.

Visit

Fast Start: The Simple 3 Step Approach

The Inner Game of Weight Loss™ has been discovered and developed from a really simple 3 step process. And it is now time to share with you the programs Fast Start.

The Introduction to The Inner Game of Weight Loss™ Fast Start is designed for us to identify your strengths, unique abilities, thinking & preferred communication styles. *Leveraging what you will become to know as the Awakened Advantage.*

Here let me ask you a question:

Would you rather focus on your strengths or focus on your weaknesses?

To say it a little different would you rather improve your strengths and have stronger strengths or would you rather improve your weaknesses and have stronger weaknesses?

1) I'd rather have Stronger Strengths

2) I'd rather have Stronger Weaknesses

(Circle your answer)

If you choose stronger strengths, that is aligned with our thinking and even my 6 year old daughters. ☺

To identify your inner game strengths we have aligned and partnered with the world class and leading authorities in assessment tools. Taking these assessments alone will Fast Start your opportunity in working with this information. These assessments identify our unique abilities, our thinking style & our preferred communication style.

The first step in this Fast Start is completing the Step 1 Examination.

Just like a doctor would never put someone in a cast without 1st doing x-rays, or a doctor would never prescribe a medication without 1st doing an examination we a simple fun process to examine and identify your unique abilities, your thinking style & your preferred communication style.

Step 2 is to then provide possible solutions, and Step 3 is implementing those solutions.

So the three step process is Examination, Solution, and Implementation.

Does this make sense?

In step 1, the examination/assessment, it can be a simple short series of 2-3 questions or it can be a much more comprehensive- thorough this process, you know--- it is really up to the individual, student athlete, parent, really up to you, in what you want. And how deep you want to go.

In solutions what we have found is that people tend to like 3 types of solutions, **a basic, an intermediate, and an advanced.** A basic is affordable-- does not take a lot of time and/or effort. If someone is not sure what they want at first because of their financial situation, if they are cautious, if they want to think about it, or simply analyze it. A basic is a great place to start.

Intermediate is for someone who is intuitive, they move forward based on that instinct. They are very intuitive, they just move forward because it makes sense.

And then there is Advanced solution. On implementation we can move forward very quickly or we can take a much longer period of time. It is really up to the individual it is up to you and your sense of URGENCY.

Please note: The Advanced is something that you typically evolve to; people are not going to start off with the advanced. People can start off at the basic or intermediate. Typically we are NOT going to start off with the advanced. The advanced will come over time.

We have arranged for you & your parent(s) to connect by phone on a 3 Way Call for 20-30 minutes.

When we talk you will walk away with a 2 page personality thinking report, including everyone on the calls preferred communication style.

It's a lot of fun! (at least a $47 Value)

To claim this Free offer schedule a call with Brian Daly at 773-574-6600

Step 1 Examination

In the next few lines we are going to look at what is it that you want to accomplish, by when, and most importantly why?

What is it that you want to accomplish?

_____

_____

_____

_____

_____

_____

_____

"The two most important days in your life are the day you were born and the day you found out why"

-Mark Twain

Your Why:

_____

_____

_____

_____

_____

_____

_____

_____

_____

_____

_____

_____

"If you do not figure out your why you will constantly be looking for an easier how to."

Here is just two questions we may have a conversation about

1. Which of these four shapes would you tend to like the most? Then 2nd then 3rd then 4th.

     1) Square _____

     2) Triangle _____

     3) Circle _____

     4) Squiggly Line _____

2. Which would cause the most frustration in any area of your life? Then 2nd then 3rd then 4th.

1) Things not done properly or in order _____

2) Not having control _____

3) Boring or not fun _____

4) If there was conflict involved _____

MENTAL TRAINING

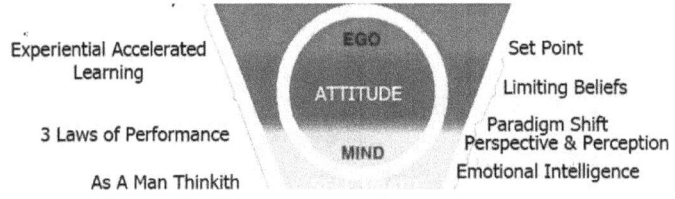

Experiential Accelerated Learning

3 Laws of Performance

As A Man Thinkith

EGO

ATTITUDE

MIND

Set Point

Limiting Beliefs

Paradigm Shift
Perspective & Perception

Emotional Intelligence

"This is your last chance. After this, there is no turning back. You take the blue pill – the story ends, you wake up in your bed and believe whatever you want to believe. You take the red pill – you stay in Wonderland and I show you how deep the rabbit-hole goes. I know you are out there. I can feel you now. I know that you're afraid of change. I don't know the future. I didn't come to tell you how this is going to end. I came here to tell you how it's going to begin."

-The Matrix Movie

IN THE GAME MINDSET

Note: This is the most important section of The Inner Game of Weight Loss™ Be sure to underline and take notes throughout this section. Again, we are laying a foundation to build on.

Let's get started with four foundational ideas.

The 1st one is the exact idea one of my coaches & mentors shared with me. It is so powerful that I want you to also write it down, right now in the space provided.:

1) "Writing is the doing part of thinking."

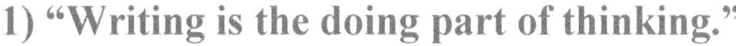

Go ahead and write the following in the space provided.
"Writing is the doing part of thinking"

If you want to make the quickest changes in your physical body, then you want to utilize the 90% of your brain that most people fail to use. To do this we **must** learn to actively engage the part of your mind through the most effective and powerful manner known today, writing.

Writing is the most hands-on and effective method of activating the part of your mind that helps you solve challenges long after you are actively thinking about them.

2) "We only see what we know."

Go ahead and write the following in the space provided.
"I only see what I know"

Steven Covey in his famous book "7 Habits of Highly Effective people" Covey introduces the concept of a paradigm shift. This chapters intention is to build on what Steven Covey brilliantly introduced to us.

The word paradigm stems from the Greek work paradeigma, originally a scientific term commonly used today to mean a perception, assumption, theory, frame of reference or lens through which we view the world.

What we see makes up our attitude: our *choice* on how we choose to view a situation, opportunity, or event.

3) "What You See Depends on Where You Are Sitting"

_____

_____

Go ahead and write the following in the space provided.
"What I See Depends On Where I am Sitting"

So how does this relate to wrestling? At some point you be given the opportunity to trust your coaches corner and perspective of a match or you are going to trust in yourself and your thoughts and feelings of how the situation occurs to you.

Rather than tell you, let me show you. What do you see below?

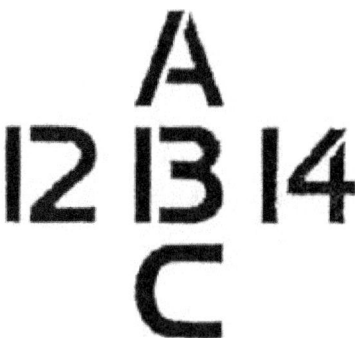

What character do you see in the uniquely arranged set of Roman letters and Arabic numerals? If we examine this horizontally first and block out the characters A and C, your brain clearly sees the sequence 12, 13 and 14.

If, however we examine this vertically and block out the numerals 12 and 14, we clearly see A, B and C. Here the context leads us to expect what we would expect to see.

Let us look at another example. What do you see below?

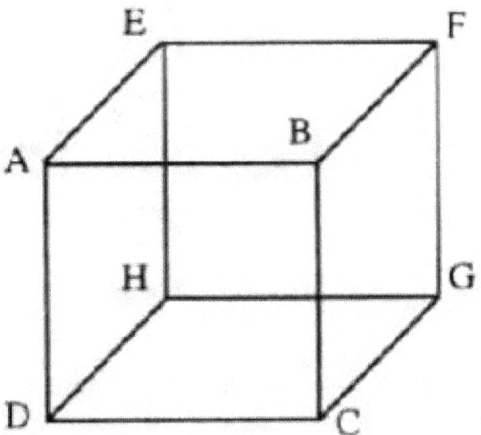

In the above visual example you will see the Necker Cube. The object below was first conceived by L.A. Necker in 1832 and is now known as the Necker Cube. It is known for its ambiguity and because it can been seen in more than one way. The Necker Cube can be seen as a cube with the face ABCD or with the face, EFGH.

"When we change the way we look at things the things we look at change"

-Wayne Dyer

4) "What You Think About Your Bring About"

Go ahead and write the following in the space provided.
"What I Think about I Bring About"

In The Inner Game of Weight Loss we practice a technique of holding one though and becoming aware of how that thought makes us feel. The longer we can focus on and hold the though and feeling of what it is we want, the greater the possibility that we get and be ready for that which we are thinking of.

What are your dominating thoughts?

What do you have your mind set on?

Below are 6 attitudes, perspectives, and/or views you can have going into a wrestling match:

1) Wrestling to Score

2) Wrestling Not to Loose

3) Wrestling to Win

4) Wrestling With An Attachment to Winning

5) Wrestling to Not Get Hurt

6) Wrestling to Pin

What is your main intention before and during your wrestling match?

So What Is Mental Toughness?

Most athletes and coaches think developing mental toughness is attained by pushing through, being focused and in the game. While it is important, it is far from the truth.

I often hear coaches say things like, be mentally tough. What does that even mean? Until creating this course the best answer I had was to push through, be ready, be focused, maybe even, pain is weakness leaving the body.

Nearly everything we do day-to-day is based on habits. Unfortunately, those habits often involve behaviors that prevent us from doing the things that lead to the next level of "success"

Being mentally tough is about building world class habits of thought.

Generally, it's about taking control of our thoughts, feelings, and attitude *before, during,* and *after* a practice and/or competition. Specifically, it is a series of being aligned and congruent with our thinking, beliefs, and behavior.

At the beginning of this program I shared with you a really great distinction of operating from a the wrong map. The map of Europe mislabeled the map of the United States. I believe this distinction has enough value that we are going to look at it once more.

Big Idea Bonus: Anytime we hear ourselves say something like "I have heard this before" it is the beginning of **hearing** what we only **listened** to the 1st time.

This happens because the 1st time we hear, read or watch something and go back to it a second time we are not the same person. We have had different experiences that have us in a different space than we were before. This is true for me since when putting together this

Inner Game of Wrestling proprietary training system I shifted as my beliefs, view and experience with the material. You can read and reread this book more than once and you will pick up new ideas that were once hidden to you.

Imagine, for a minute that you were handed a map of "Europe" and it is mislabeled the "United States."

So here we are in the United States with a map that we think is of the United States and it really is a map of Europe. Now imagine with this map of Europe we are "trying" to get to Chicago from New Jersey.

With this map as our guide would we ever be able to get from where we are to where we want to go?

With this map as our reference, would WORKING HARDER make any difference in getting us from Chicago to New Jersey?

With this map as our reference would having more FOCUS help us in getting from Chicago to New Jersey.

With this map as our reference, would spending more TIME "trying" to figure out directions make any difference?

Clearly no. Right?

Learning another take down, working on another turn from top, or an escape from bottom would be like, in this example (*again with the wrong map)* choosing to take a bike rather than walking, or deciding to drive a car rather than taking a bike. You can see how using another vehicle such as a bike or car would only get us lost even faster. Technique is really important and it is not the only variable in our highest potential.

Being motivated is not the answer because we would still be operating from the wrong map. It would just get us lost even faster leaving us even more frustrated.

Being more focused, working harder and longer, being stronger and faster is not always the solution.

One solution is: To stop and ask someone who has been there before to train us and teach us that this is a map of Europe and not a map of the United States."

Our mindset is our belief systems.

Our belief system is our map.

Mental toughness is developing a new view the world, ourselves, and others. Shifting our view paradigm, or map of what we believe is possible.

"Do not conform to the pattern of this world, but be transformed by the renewing of your mind"

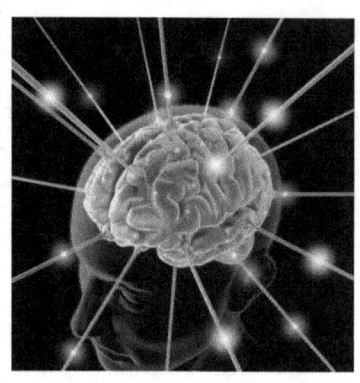

<u>In Fact</u>: In the past 8 years alone, we have learned so much about the power of the brain that literally 80% to 90% of what we thought we knew before is now obsolete.

In scientific terms, our mind is divided into the conscious mind and the subconscious mind.

The function of our conscious mind is reason, memory, perception, imagination and intuition. To do this, our conscious mind uses our five senses of taste, touch, smell, sight, and sound. Expanding our awareness through these senses is critical to accessing the Power of Now!

The function of our subconscious mind acts as our personal operating system. Yes, you have your own, Apple IOS and/or Android operating system.

It is said that our subconscious mind controls a miraculous 96-98% of all our perception and behaviors. This system stores our beliefs and memories as well as connects us to the Lord. God, Infinite Intelligence. This is the powerhouse, which filters and conditions our beliefs, attitudes, feelings, emotions, and memories. It runs like a program.

As your program is always running, look at these ideas, compare, test, and observe these relationships and we will often see something that you did not see before.

Think of it like a temperature thermostat on the wall. Our "personal thermostat" to notify us of changes. Our thermostat controls keeping us safe, away from threats and comfortable. We now know that when the brain subconsciously holds us back, it actually thinks that it is doing its job by keeping us safe within in our map of reality.

You have a subconscious belief system that operates like a map. When we test something outside of this belief system our mind feels threatened and it "protects" us.

The good news is that as this is happening, our brain is hardwired and responsible for looking for connections, filtering, filing and organizing moments and processing data, alerting us of what's important to pay attention to.

The most important aspect of the subconscious mind is that it does not know the difference between what is real and what is imagined. It believes whatever we continue to impress upon it.

We have a proven process, which is made up of the use of triggers and emotions to create a clear vision of intent. We can imprinting our vision into the subconscious powerhouse of our mind. Once this image and idea is chosen and consistently impressed WITH EMOTION into the subconscious mind, perceptions and behaviors change to find and produce the desire result. Think the movie: Inception.

Let's look at what happens in our brain when we visualize the future. There are two parts of our brain, the conscious and subconscious. The conscious part is the part that we are aware of, typically -- we think of it as the "me" that does the thinking. That's because the conscious brain focuses on one thing at a time (whatever we think is most important at that moment) and constructs logical sequences: "If I do this, then this will happen, and then that." The subconscious doesn't think this way; it sees a complete picture of everything happening all at once.

Think of it this way. The subconscious mind is aware of the input from all of your senses at every moment. Every inch of your skin is sending it information right now but for the most part, your conscious mind only becomes aware of it if it is alerted that something needs its attention. That's the whole purpose of pain in fact. That's the subconscious mind's way of getting the conscious mind's attention to something that is a danger or is damaging the body. Because the subconscious mind can only do what has been done before. It needs the conscious mind to "think outside the box." But in order for the conscious mind to do its job, it needs the subconscious mind to take care of everything else.

When most people think of intelligence, they think of the conscious brain functions. After all, it is the crown jewel of human development. Through its brilliant capacity for imagination, it can soar throughout the universe; through its astonishing faculties of logic, reason, and analysis, it can learn, invent, design, and grasp a staggering range of phenomena. However, it only represents only a tiny fraction of the whole brain's function. The amount of information your conscious brain processes is about one-half of one-millionth of one percent of the amount your subconscious brain processes!

For all its brilliance, the conscious brain has a major weakness; follow-through. The conscious brain is great at imagining things and thinking them through, but it's next to useless when it comes to actually getting things done.

The conscious mind is like the writer-director of a film. It can write a brilliant screenplay, but until you bring in set designers, costumers, carpenters, sound engineers, electricians, makeup people, composers and musicians, editors, and, of course, a full complement of actors to carry out the story, all you have is words on a page. And it's your subconscious brain that carries out all the functions of every one of those hundreds and thousands of other roles.

So why is your conscious brain amazing at coming up with an idea but useless when it comes to actually carrying it out? Because it is easily distracted. The average person changes focus every six to ten seconds; the conscious brain has to struggle to remember more than three or four things at a time. On the other hand, the subconscious can remember billions of things in perfect sequence, not only for minutes at a time but for your entire lifetime. And, how often does it get distracted? *Never.* It is absolutely astounding there are some ten quadrillion different biochemical processes happening in your body every second—and your subconscious is keeping track of all of them.

So let me ask you, which part of your brain would you want to trust to deliver on your wrestling dream: the part that has trouble staying focused and remembering a phone number, or the part than runs quadrillions of complex biochemical processes at the same time, twenty four hours a day, every day of your life?

THE POWER OF WORDS

Now I have to warn you 1st this gets a deep.

The problem & opportunity here is that from birth language is given to us. It is not that we learn language, language is here waiting for us.

My favorite book says "In the beginning was the Word , and the Word was with God, and the Word was God."

So much of life exists in language and communication. And many of us have a weak relationship with the power and meaning behind the words that we choose and how we can be conditioned by it.

We are being hypnotized by the destructive music we listen to.

Here let me explain, before competition while warming up before EVERY match I listed to "I Tried" by Bone Thugs & Harmony. Knowing what I know now there may NOT be a worse song of lyrics to expose my subconscious mind to prior to competition.

Here read the chorus below, and aside from the beat determine for yourself if the words are empowering or disempowering.

"I Tried" (by Akon)

You know nothing come easy, you **gotta try real real hard, I tried hard...but I guess I gotta try harder.**

[Chorus]

I try so hard **can't seem to get away from misery**
man I try so hard **will always be a victim** of these streets **it ain't my fault** cause I...tried to get away but trouble follows me and **still I try so hard** hoping one day you'll come and rescue me **but until then, I'll be posted up right here rain sleet hail snow but until then... I'll be posted up right here with my heat getting dough**

[Verse]

It's like **I'm taking 5 steps forward and 10 steps back, trying to get ahead of the game,** but I **can't seem to get it on track**, and I keep running away from the ones that say they love me the most how could I create the distance when it's suppose to be close and uh, I just don't know but I be out here fighting demons and, **it's like a curse that I can't shake** this part of Cleveland and lord, would you help me? and stop this pain I keep inflicting on my family hustling gambling, tricking and scamming scrambling and losing sight of what I'm suppose to be handling, it's hard to manage **cause everyday's a challenge** and man I'm slipping can't lose my balance I'm trying not to panic

[Chorus (Akon)]

I try so hard **can't seem to get away from misery**
man I try so hard **will always be a victim** of these streets it ain't my fault cause I... tried to get away but trouble follows me
and still **I try so hard** hoping one day you'll come and rescue me
but until then, I'll be posted up right here rain sleet hail snow but until then... I'll be posted up right here with my heat getting dough

Please stop using the word "try." Trying implies failure. There is actually no state of trying.

The word "Try" is a poorly programmed word because try implies failure. Again there is no state of trying. We either do something or we do not.

Here, let me give you a real example. Take out a pen, your keys, something, and throw it out onto the floor. Go ahead, do it. Throw it on the floor.

Ok, now "try" to pick it up. "Try" to pick it up. You see, either you pick it up or you do not. When we say we are going to "try" and do something we actually give ourselves a REASON for not accomplishing what you set out to do.

At the end, when you do not get to result we set out for we say, well I "tried."

The 1st step is becoming aware (conscious) that this is happening, weather you realize it or not. Then and only then do we have the power of choice.

We can choose to either be at the effect and influenced by what we are allowing into our mind or be in control of what we allow to be spoken over our life.

Here is why our words have such a significant impact on our physical body and the physical world. When we use a word we encode meaning and a picture with that word. The words we use consistently make up the fabric of our thought and thoughts become things. Remember:

"What You Think About Your Bring About"

Many of us have a weak relationship with the true meaning behind the words that we choose. What naturally holds us back is our poor relationship with language.

It is not so much the words that we use but our associations with this words, the meaning we give to the words.

Non-supportive, subconscious beliefs are created and further developed from people in our life, the environment and the "world"

The following are **6 Low Value Words** that that you may want to consider replacing with High Value Words to experience more confidence, and clarity:

1. **Try…..** Try is a poorly programmed word because try implies failure. There is actually no state of trying. Either you do something **or** you do not. Here, I will prove it to you. Take the pen that you are using to take notes in this Course and throw it on the floor. Go ahead; throw it on the floor now. Ok, now try to pick it up. Try to pick it up. You see, you either pick it up or you do not. The word "try" actually gives you a reason for not accomplishing what you set yourself out to do. At the end, when you do not get to the goal you say, "I tried."

2. **Can't…..** When we use the word "can't," what we are really saying is either "I do not know how to"; or "I do not want to." The same goes for when someone else uses the word "can't." What they are actually saying is, "I do not know how to"; or "I do not want to." Instead, stop yourself when you hear yourself use the word "<u>can't</u>"; and ask yourself, "Is it that I do not know how to"; or "Is it that I do not want to?" Same goes for when someone tells you they can't do something. To clear up this communication, challenge the other person by asking, "Is it that you do not know how to do what I'm asking?" or "Do you just not want to?" The reason for not being able to because of not knowing is entirely different that not being able to because of not wanting to.

3. **But…..** "But" is a non-supportive programming word because it neglects or disregards everything before it. For example: "We played well, <u>but</u> we still lost." What is actually

being said at a deep subconscious level is, "We did not play well." The right way to reprogram yourself is to replace "but" with "and." So, the same statement would be: "We played well and still lost." Anywhere that we use the word "but," we can replace it with "and." Using this technique affirms, gives strength, and truth to the first part of the statement.

4. **Hope**....Hope as a verb or action is a non-supportive programming word because it implies lack of knowing. For example, see the subtle difference in the following: "I hope we perform at our best tomorrow" compared to, "I know we will perform at our best tomorrow." The second example, at a deep subconscious level, removes all negative non-supportive programming. So, instead of using the word "hope," replace it with "know."

5. **If**.....is a terrible programming word because it also implies lack of knowing, faith, and confidence. Instead, remove the word <u>if</u> from your language and replace it with "when." See the difference in the following example? "If we win tonight, we are going for pizza afterwards" compared to "When we win tonight, we are going for pizza." These last two examples in #4 and #5 both follow the principle of "Always beginning with the end in mind."

6. **Problem**..... is a useless programming word because it implies doubt or difficulty. We can always replace the perceived obstacle as an "Opportunity" or a "Challenge." Let me clarify. Do you really want any more problems in your life? Or, do you like to be challenged? Or, be presented with an opportunity?

These 6 Low Value Words are just a few to make the point that there is so much power in language. You now have the first step two steps in developing a winning attitude, your awareness and communication.

My challenge to you now is to become aware of how often you use one or all of these words and be responsible with now knowing the impact.

Again, this will develop more and more as you reflect on what you've learned in this Book and allow your subconscious mind to make even deeper connections.

Introducing….The Lifestyle Triangle

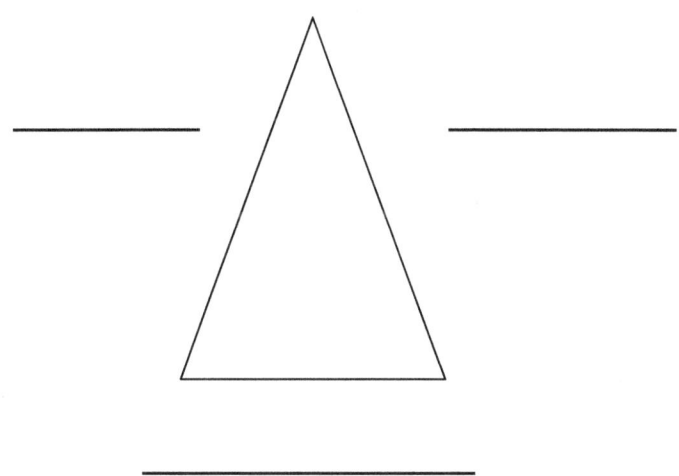

(Sorry this is only available to those in The Inner Game of Weight Loss Team)

Step 2) Possible Solutions

You can now start to see the genius of tapping in to this powerhouse, can't you? With all that we have shared with you, you have an opportunity to, in a moment, make a decision.

Now knowing this new information, are you going to continue doing things the old way, the hard way? **or** *Do you want to commit to and decide to leverage your untapped potential leveraging this latest scientific research?*

If you made the decision to use this new information, I acknowledge you for being open to the coaching. Now, if you want to move through the program faster, and/or get an experience of personally working with Brian & his team. You have 1 of 2 options.

Option 1:
You keep doing what you are doing, taking on the RISK of wasting time, energy and resources to still NOT get the end result you want.

If not this, what will you do differently this season?

_____
_____
_____
_____
_____
_____
_____
_____
_____

Option 2:
You Now Take Action and Click or Call to Apply to The Inner Game of Weight Loss™ Team.

Either way it really is just a decision. And remember no decision is still a decision.

Step 3 Action

To Apply to The Inner Game of Weight Loss™ Team.

Visit
or Call 773-574-6600

SPIRITUAL TRAINING

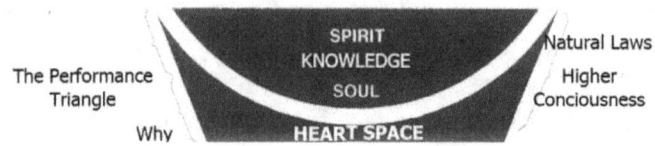

"Our deepest fear is not that we are inadequate. Our deepest fear is that we are powerful beyond imagination. It is our light more than our darkness which scares us.

We ask ourselves – who are we to be brilliant, beautiful, talented, and fabulous. But honestly, who are you to not be so?

You are a child of God, small games do not work in this world. For those around us to feel peace, it is not example to make ourselves small. We were born to express the glory of God that lives in us. It is not in some of us, it is in all of us.

While we allow our light to shine, we unconsciously give permission for others to do the same. When we liberate ourselves from our own fears, simply our presence may liberate others."

Marianne Williamson
In Return to Love
Nelson Mandela's Inaugural Address
The Movie Coach Carter

The Inner Game of Weight Loss program is heavy on **Knowledge** & **Attitude.** The Skills of Wrestling can be taught from any qualified coach who has completed at a high level. And there are more than enough technicians to teach you these physical skills: setups, take downs and go to wrestling moves.

When I 1st discovered the image that this program is design off of I couldn't believe it. When looking closely at it, working with it, testing it, everything I thought to be true about wrestling performance was flipped upside down.

I saw what I couldn't see before, how strengthening our spirit makes so much sense for wrestling and life.

I mean in wrestling...

One of our main goals is to break the other wrestler's spirit or will to go on. So why do we only focus on physical training?

The absolute bestselling book of all time says "physical training is of some value, but godliness has value for all things, holding promise for both the present life and the life to come."

Another great message from the book declares: "For we wrestle not against flesh and blood, but against principalities, against powers, against the rulers of the darkness of this world, against spiritual wickedness in high places."

So who are the principalities, what kind of powers are we talking about, who are these rulers of the darkness of this world and who are these spiritually wicked in high places?

Well before we can deal with this enemy we 1st have to define who this enemy is.

This enemy is also known as resistance. Steven Pressfield in his easy read book The War of Art did a great job of defining this enemy RESISTANCE. Pressfield shares "Resistance cannot be seen, touched, heard or smelled, but it can be felt. It's a repelling force. Its negative, Its aim is to shove us away, distract us, prevent us from doing our work."

Pressfield continues "Resistance seems to come from outside ourselves and arises within".

Recommended Reading: "The War of Art" by Steven Pressfield

Now that we have identified this enemy let's look at the enemies plan. One of my favorite books says "The thief comes only to steal, kill, and destroy"

Just like black is to white, and day is to night, the contrast to resistance is assistance. And we can find our assistance in someone. Someone who is for us and not against us. A light in this dark world. The leader amongst leaders.

The good news is that this enemy operates under the authority of Christ. And needs permission to tempt and test us.

Spiritual performance is learning to let go and lean on God for strength. Giving up our perspective, our view and our understanding of things.

My favorite book declares "Turning your ear to wisdom and applying your heart to understanding."

Wisdom is really execution of knowledge. What we know to do.

Whoever said that knowledge is power is an idiot. Knowledge is NOT power. Power is having all the right information at the given time to choose to take action, influence and produce results

I am still learning to distinguish which battles are for us to fight and which are for Him to fight. And He says 'Not by might nor by power, but by my Spirit,' says the Lord Almighty.

Here is a short prayer to support us in doing this:

God, grant me the serenity to accept the things I cannot change, The courage to change the things I can, And the wisdom to know the difference.

You see a few years after missing the mark at the NCAA National Championships I had an undeniable experience with Christ. A transformation. I came to the conclusion that throughout my wrestling career I trusted too much on my own talent, strengths, and abilities.

I discovered a relationship with Christ. Not religion but relationship. A new perspective on life. Sure I wrestled with this new truth as you might as well and have decided in my heart that there is a God, He is for us and we have the choice to acknowledge, accept and receiving Jesus into our hearts.

It is a choice.

I challenge you to find what is true for you. "Ask, and it shall be given you; seek, and ye shall find; knock, and it shall be opened unto you."

And yes it takes faith. "Faith is being sure of what we hope for and certain of what we do not see"

Faith in Action: My favorite book put declares it this way "You see that his faith and his actions were working together, and his faith was made complete by what he did"

An Awakened Athlete™ trains not only for physical performance but also trains for mental and spiritual performance. Working on the 3 things that matter: training our mind, training our body and training our spirit.

Each of these three relationships are shown below, with the three overlapping circles. They reveal how each area independently, as well as together, connect and work together for an Awakened Athlete.

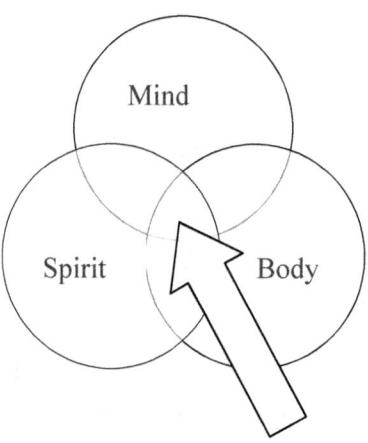

Awakened Advantage

The center of the diagram shows the "sweet spot" that makes up our Awakened Advantage.

We train and develop this advantage over our competition with the only three things that can be learned and taught.

Record these three definitions:

Knowledge: Applied information X's (times) your experiences.

Attitude: Mindset, Beliefs

Skill: A learned behavior and/or developed competency.

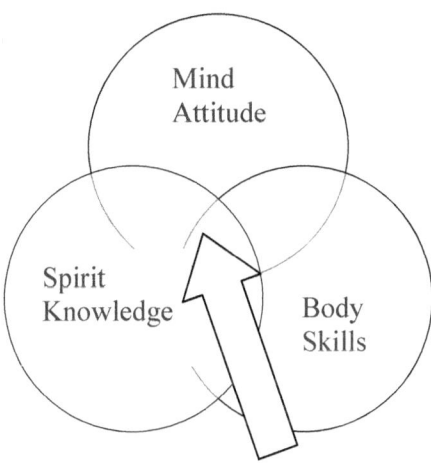

Awakened Advantage

PHYSICAL TRAINING

This book is NOT focused on the technique of wrestling: setups, take downs and moves.. There are more than enough technicians and wrestling camps for this type of training.

All skillsets are learnable.

Skillsets are learned behavior.

The Skillsets to The Inner Game of Weight Loss™ are determined by your ability to reflect on ideas of this program and ask the question "how can this apply ro me?" And then turn that into an action. And consistently take that action enough times.

So how long do we have to work at something before we get good at it?

Malcolm Gladwell in his bestselling book Outliers shares many examples of the "10,000-Hour Rule", physiologists in the expertise research field concluded the key to "success" in any field is, to a large extent, a matter of practicing a specific task for a total of around 10,000 hours. So at 4 hours a day mastery is about 10 years.

Well what if we do not have 10 years?

Great question.

EXPERIENTIAL ACCELERATED LEARNING

Experiential Accelerated Learning is shortening time with learning by doing.

In order to accelerate our learning curve, we can speed up the process by following time-tested laws, principles, and most important the latest scientific research. As we stressed before, **knowledge without immediate action is just like not knowing.**

Note: The application & action is where the game is won and/or lost.

Below is a copy of the diagram by Edgar Dale. At the turn of the century educationist Edgar Dale illustrated how people can very quickly learn a new skill and he illustrated this with an image "The Cone of Learning"

It shows the benefits of active learning over passive learning.

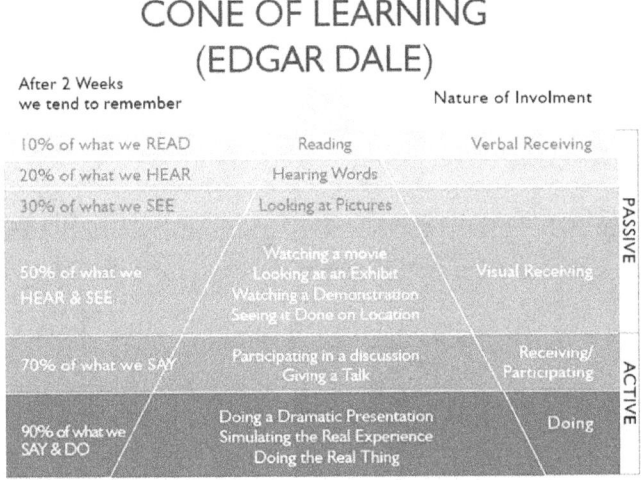

According to Dale's research, after two weeks we remember only 10% of what we read, but remember 90% of what we take action on or do." (You can also Google this).

Here is the problem with this book, if 70% of people read 30% of a book and Cone of Learning diagram tells us that we only remember 10% of what we read, We are only really retaining 10% of 30% of the material. That is only 3% of the information.

The point here is that our performance results will NOT come from learning ABOUT The Inner Game of Weight Loss™ from a book, it will come from you seeing value in it and having an experience with this technology and APPLYING it.

The cone charts the average retention rate for various methods of teaching. The further you progress down the cone, the greater the learning and the more information is likely to be retained

It reveals that "action-learning" techniques result in up to 90% retention. People learn best when they use perceptual learning styles. Perceptual learning styles are sensory based. The more sensory channels possible in interacting with a resource, the better chance that many students can learn from it.

His research led to the development of the Cone of Experience. Today, this "learning by doing" has become known as "experiential learning" or "action learning".

The "4 Laws of Learning"

To take this a step further, Experiential Accelerated Learning is based in the 4 Laws of Learning which are:

1. Unconscious Incompetence

2. Consciously Incompetence

3. Unconscious Competence

4. Consciously Competence

In this Inner Game of Weight Loss program, we look at and use these Four Levels of Learning to identify where we are at in the process of being competent with a developed skillset. Competent here means, having the necessary ability, knowledge, or skill to do something efficient. Being capable.

Law 1: The Law of Unconscious Incompetence

Here is the thing, there are natural laws work for us and against us. And they really work for us when we become present to them and the impact they have.

The Law of Unconscious Incompetence states: *we don't know something and we don't know that we don't know.*

To get past this unconscious level we must become aware. The goal here is to examine where we are and move through to Level 4.

For example a wrestler might be a competent wrestler and a incompetent coach. Why? Often great wrestlers are not aware of what they do to be great. They are unconscious, meaning performance is occur automatically or unconsciously competent.

To get past this unconscious level we must become awakened to information just like this.

Law 2: Pareto Law or the Law of 80/20:

Pareto Law states that 80% of our results come from 20% of our effort.

So if you are asking yourself what are the 20% of actions will give me the 80% of the results I want? Great question...

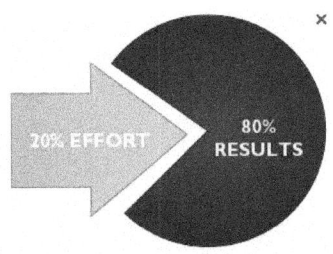

Effective training is using the Law of 80/20 to maximize our training efforts. This includes our ability to consistently train at peak levels and stay injury free.

One of the best ways to stay injury free is to train using high intensity low duration training; measuring, when possible our heart rate zones to guarantee we are maximizing every workout, our time and energy.

Introducing... A New Training Model

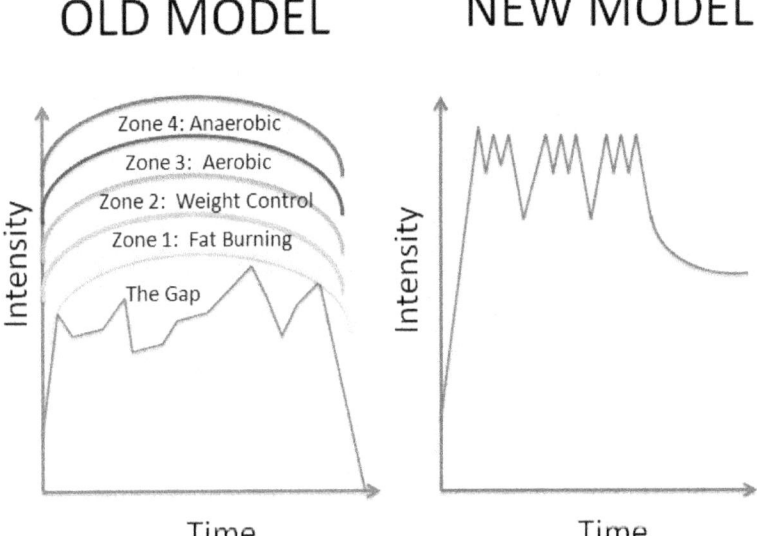

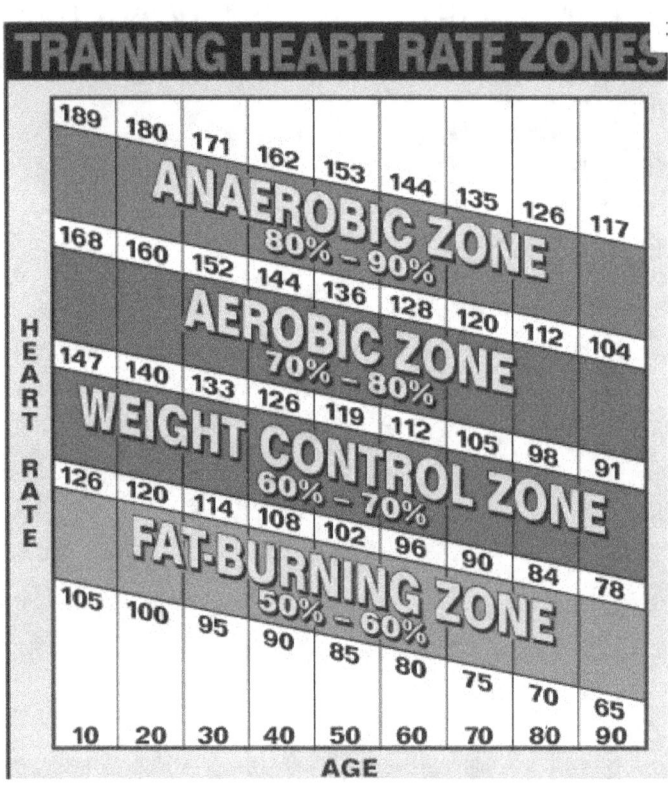

Here is why you should care about your heart rate?

The Distinction #5:
Aerobic vs Anaerobic

Aerobic exercise builds health & burns fat.
(180- age) = Minimum Heart Rate
Aerobic means "with oxygen"
When we condition our metabolism
To operate aerobically and supply it with proper diet and exercise you
burn fat as your primary fuel.

Anaerobic exercise builds muscle.
(220- your age) = Max Heart Rate
Anaerobic means "without oxygen"
Anaerobic exercise burns glycogen (sugar) as its primary fuel, while causing the body to store fat.

What do you want to focus on? (The % is of your Maximum Heart Rate)
A. Fat Burning 50-60%
B. Weight Control 60-70%
C. Aerobic 70-80%
D. Anaerobic 80-90%

An Introduction to Entrepreneurship

"The pursuit of opportunity without regard to resources currently controlled"

Vision: A Life Focus

The world's all time bestselling book ever says" "Without a vision the people perish"

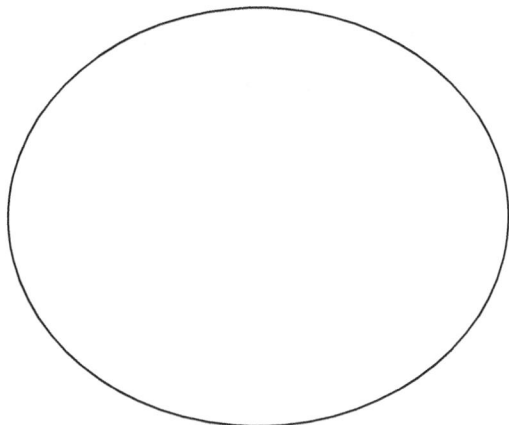

Please ask your Inner Game of Wrestling Mentor to walk you through this above circle, it's really cool and only takes really 11 minutes or less.

This is the same process I went through to find and believe my Life Focus. I believe that my life purpose is to develop teams, train, & serve wrestlers & work with entrepreneurs. Sharing the skillset of Entrepreneurship, Business, and Opportunity.

If you are still reading this I want you to send me a text right now to 773-574-6600. Yes this paragraph is a test to see if you are still with me.

What I just can't wrap my head around is, why is it that we "invest" our parents invest in our education for at least 17 years of education from kindergarten to 8th Grade (9 years), High School (4 Years), and College, (lucky to complete in 4 Years), before we hope to apply what we have learned in those 17 years of school or more to only then start to earn a living and make a return on our investment.

I don't know of an investor who would wait 17 years for a return on their money. When we look at this through this perspective, why are we still thinking that the one thing standing in our way of our success is a fancy College MBA? Is the model of going to school to then get a good, safe job afterwards broken?

"School teaches us how to gather information, entrepreneurship teaches us how to apply it to make a living"

A possible solution: Entrepreneurship
Below are the 3 different styles of Entrepreneurship

1) Social Entrepreneur
2) Serial Entrepreneur
3) Lifestyle Entrepreneur

Social Entrepreneur

A Social Entrepreneur is motivated by a desire to help, improve and transform social, environmental, educational and economic conditions. Key traits and characteristics of highly effective social entrepreneurs include ambition and a lack of acceptance of the status quo or accepting the world "as it is". The social entrepreneur is driven by an emotional desire to address some of the big social and economic conditions in the world, for example, poverty and educational rather than by the desire for profit. Social entrepreneurs seek to develop innovative solutions to global problems that can be copied by others to enact change.

Social entrepreneurs act within a market aiming to create social value through the improvement of goods and services offered to the community. Their main aim is to help offer a better service -- improving the community as a whole.

Serial Entrepreneur

A serial entrepreneur is continuously comes up with new ideas and starts new businesses. As opposed to a typical entrepreneur who will often come up with an idea, start the company and then see it through and play an important role in the day functioning of the new company, a serial entrepreneur will often come up with the idea and get things started, but then give responsibility to someone else and move on to a new idea and a new venture. This can be a good thing if the individual has lots of unique ideas and is the best one suited to get each one started, but can be a bad thing if the individual stops putting time into a company that needs his or her help, in order to move forward with a new idea that may or may not succeed.

Lifestyle Entrepreneur

A lifestyle entrepreneur places passion before profit when launching a business in order to combine personal interests and talent with the ability to earn a living. Many entrepreneurs may be primarily motivated by the intention to make their business profitable in order to sell to shareholders. In contrast, a lifestyle entrepreneur intentionally chooses a business model intended to develop and grow their business in order to make a long-term, sustainable and viable living, working in a field where they have a particular interest, passion, talent, knowledge or high degree of expertise. A lifestyle entrepreneur may decide to become self-employed in order to achieve greater personal freedom, more family time and more time working on projects or business goals that inspire them. A lifestyle entrepreneur may combine a hobby with a profession or they may specifically decide not to expand their business in order to remain in control of their venture. Common goals held by the lifestyle entrepreneur include earning a living doing something that they love, earning a living in a way that facilitates self-employment, achieving a good work balance and owning a business without shareholders. Many lifestyle entrepreneurs are very dedicated to their business and may work within the creative industries where a passion before profit approach to entrepreneurship often prevails. While many entrepreneurs may launch their business with a clear exit strategy a lifestyle entrepreneur may deliberately and consciously choose to keep their venture fully within their own control. Lifestyle entrepreneurship is increasing popular as technology provides small business with the digital platforms needed to reach a large global market.

Which of the 3 styles of Entrepreneurship resonates with you, write it below in the space provided.

_____

Introducing... "Easy Entrepreneurship"

Product	Market	Cost
Service	List	Offer
Experience	Distribution	Agreement

As you can see this image is divided into three categories. The market makes up all the products, services and experiences people are willing and able to purchase.

Distribution is the process by which we are going to deliver the product, service or experience to the customer.

A smart way to think of the List & Distribution Distinction is to ask: "Who already offers or sells products, services or experiences to my ideal customer?" When we figure out who is already offering products, services and experiences to the same customers we are looking to reach we can partner up to offer these same customers something else. Of course there needs to be an incentive for whoever is providing the distribution or the list of customers. This is known as a joint venture.

For now let's stay with The Easy Entrepreneur Distinction. When we know the **Total Cost** of the creation, marketing, & delivery of the product, service and/or experience we can then and only then come up with a price to test and see if people are willing & able to exchange that life energy for the product, experience, or service.

Here let me explain more: When we know the Total Cost or in other terms the Total Cost to Acquire a Customer we then know how much we can afford to pay to acquire a new customer. **Then and only then do we have a real business.** (When we know the Cost to Acquire a Customer)

To take it one step further we can determine the Initial Value of that Customer & then determine the Lifetime Value of that Customer. How much that customer is worth to us initially and then how much that customer is worth over the lifetime of the customer doing business with us. This information is important in understanding how much we can spend in providing that customer an amazing experience with us. Pretty straight forward, right.

Creating Offers and Using Agreements

Creating & designing an attractive, high converting offer means an offer where the value of the offer is easy to get, clear and easy to say yes to. Meeting the needs of people. The bigger the problem and the pain we solve the larger the reward and payoff for us.

When creating a great offer, we look from The 3 P's of an Irresistible Offer: Positioning, Packaging, & Promoting.

Before we promote our offer to the market we want to do our research and study what people are already purchasing, where are they buying it, and from who are they purchasing and for what price.

Each product, service or experience is meeting some need in which people are looking to get met.
Knowing this information allows us the opportunity to differentiate ourselves and position our marketing message in the market, with our advantage. Positioning our message against any perceived "competition."

Of the 3 P's to and Irresistible Offer, Positioning is the most important. Positing & Packaging also includes having a combination of both a strong branding & direct response marketing.

For me Entrepreneurship can be summarized as finding and solving someone's specific problem, show that we have the solution and create an agreement that with specific deal points, promises, terms and deliverables.

One of the best ways to understand what's possible with agreements is to look from the contracts that are included on the next page.

Note: Agreements are made through relationships. Having these contracts mean nothing unless we understand how to clearly communicate our ideas.

These are the exact contracts we use to take advantage of opportunities. They will need to be edited per deal and include deal points.

The Only 3 Ways to Grow a Business

There are 3 ways and only 3 ways to grow a business.

1) Getting More Customers
2) Increase the Transaction Size
3) Increase the Frequency of Purchase

And inside these only 3 ways to grow there are some very specific strategies.

This book is intended to be an introduction to small business & entrepreneurship. If you have a business and/or want one, get with the author and/or visit www.3DayMBAbook.com

JOINT VENTURE AGREEMENT

JOINT VENTURE LICENSE AGREEMENT

JOINT VENTURE CO-DEVELOPMENT AGREEMENT

LICENSE AGREEMENT

MARKETING AGREEMENT

PROMOTIONAL PARTNER & PARTNERSHIP AGREEMENT

BUY/SELL SHAREHOLDER AGREEMENT

DISTRIBUTOR AGREEMENT

MARKETING AND DISTRIBUTION AGREEMENT

ROYALTY AGREEMENT

CONSULTING AGREEMENT

HOURLY CONSULTING AGREEMENT

MONTHLY RETAINER COPYWRITING AND CONSULTING AGREEMENT

COPYWRITING AGREEMENT& COPYWRITING AND REVENUE SHARING AGREEMENT

LICENSE AND ROYALTY AGREEMENT

LIST USAGE AGREEMENT

LOAN AND INVESTMENT AGREEMENT & RELEASE

Final Note

Even though I lost out on being an All American, I believe that a pain is never wasted. There is so much value in our life experiences and we now use this knowledge to help wrestlers just like you.

We are now able to reach even more coaches and parents who are joining in on the movement to give their kids access to the best resources and opportunities available.

Although my search started outside of myself, I ended up with an awakening within. One that completely changed my view on peak performance. The ultimate answers were within.

I want to leave you with one final definition. This definition is the definition of insanity. Insanity is doing the same thing over and over again and expecting a different result. And forget the idea that you need to practice more, work harder and longer—be stronger & faster. It didn't work for me and by now it should be clear that it is not the answer.

So in a moment I am going to ask you to very specifically write what it is you are going to do differently this season and/or off season.

What will you do differently this year?

_____

_____

_____

_____

_____

_____

_____

_____

_____

I have purposely kept this Inner Game of Weight Loss short because as statistics tell us you probably haven't even read this far into the book.

The biggest mistake you can make after reading this is to move back into the idea of "practice makes perfect."

To ensure this does not happen, you should make certain that you follow the most powerful principles as you read to engage your subconscious mind. (If you do not, remember to re-read this The Inner Game of Weight Loss™ immediately.)

Please Do Not Read The Following Summary Points Until You Have Read This 3 Times...

I trust that if you are now reading this section that you have worked through this book three times or have taken advantage of one of our offers with one of our coaches.

By now, I trust that you have seen the genius of The Inner Game of Weight Loss. By now, you should have an idea of its value to you.

If you are ready to continue to challenge your assumptions about "success," and are your ready to experience the power of making sure your using the right map I challenge you to take action and apply for our Inner Game of Wrestling Team.

We look forward to personally working with you and challenging what you think is possible.

To your greatness,

Brian Daly

Inner Game of Weigh Loss™ Agreement

CoCreated with You & Your Mentor

The following agreement made on _____ of_____ 2015
between Brian Daly, _____ (Student Athlete)
and_____. (Parent)

Parent Signature _____

Student Signature _____

Application Approval Signature _____

The Inner Game of Weight Loss™

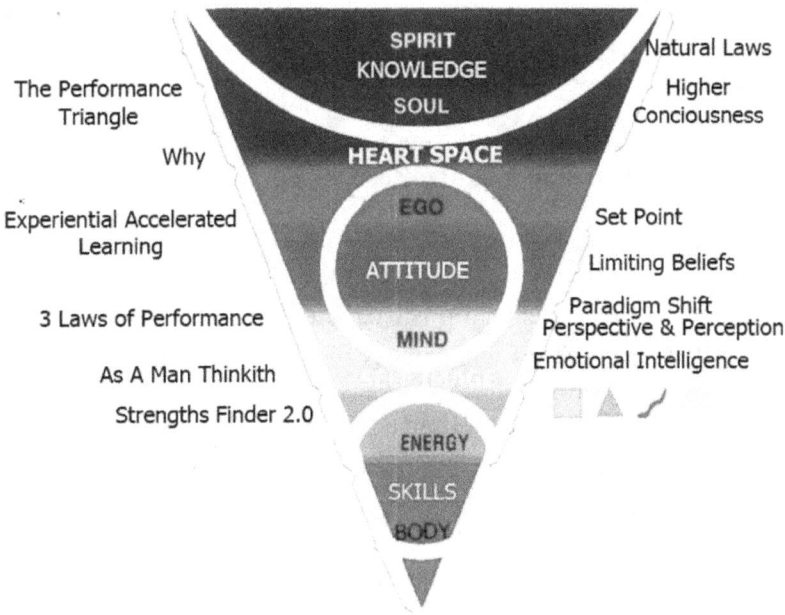

Intention:

To Develop You the Leader Within You

Outcomes:

1. You will experience a positive winning culture that causes you to stretch your vision of what's possible.

2. You will know yourself as a leader, with an increase in confidence and the ability to trust your training in the moments that matter most.

3. You will breakthrough any limiting beliefs that are holding you back.

☐ Yes Brian, I am choosing to do something different this year .

I am NOW making a 6 month commitment to you, and myself. I am deciding to follow your process and I am coachable.

Student Athlete: _____

Parents Name: _____

Address:_____

City: _____ State: _____ Zip:_____

E-mail*: _____

Phone: _____

Credit Card: (check one)
Visa: _____ MasterCard: _____ Other: _____

3 Digit Code: _____

Amount Today $_____

Credit Card Number: _____

Exp. Date: _____

Signature: _____

Date: _____

*Providing this information constitutes your permission for The Inner Game of Weight Loss
to contact you regarding related information via mail, e-mail, fax, and phone

About The Author:

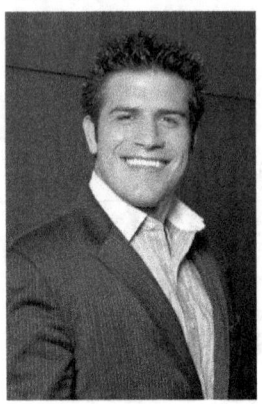

Brian Daly Entrepreneur, Author & Founder & Lead Coach at The Inner Game of Weight Loss™.

For close to a decade, Brian competed as a top Nationally-Ranked Wrestler, where he competed 4x's at the NCAA National Championships, was invited 2x's to the largest Division I NCAA Championship Tournament, and received the U.S. Marine Corp Award.

These may seem like great accomplishments for any individual, however Brian saw it differently. Each and every year for 7 years straight, he qualified for the High School State and College NCAA National Championships. And each and every year, Brian was unable to achieve his goal of being an All-American or National Champion. When it came down to the most critical moments of competition, there was always something that just seemed to happen, leaving Brian disappointed and with many unanswered questions.

Brian's purpose in life is to work with wrestlers and develop their leadership, a positive mental attitude & expose them to the possibilities of being an Entrepreneur. He believes being an entrepreneur is the solution to the challenges with the current educations system.

Brian a Coach, Entrepreneur & Author of 2 Books, **"The Inner Game of Weight Loss™"** & **"3 Day MBA"** Everything You Will Never Get From Business School www.3DayMBABook.com

Brian currently lives in Chicago, IL near Midway Airport and married to his beautiful wife Francielle, has two girls, 6 year old daughter Nelyssa and new born baby girl Genesis.

Request a Free 3 Way 30 Minute Strategy Session. Many times this call looks like a call between you and our leadership team.

To Schedule a time that works for everyone Call 773-574-6600.

Or To Apply to The Inner Game of Weight Loss™ Team.

Visit

BONUS:

AS A MAN THINKETH

BY JAMES ALLEN

Mind is the Master power that moulds and makes,

And Man is Mind, and evermore he takes

The tool of Thought, and, shaping what he wills,

Brings forth a thousand joys, a thousand ills:

He thinks in secret, and it comes to pass:

Environment is but his looking glass.

Authorized Edition

Public Domain, New York

CONTENTS

THIS little volume (the result of meditation and experience) is not intended as an exhaustive treatise on the much written upon subject of the power of thought. It is suggestive rather than explanatory, its object being to stimulate men and women to the discovery and perception of the truth that

"They themselves are makers of themselves."by virtue of the thoughts, which they choose and encourage; that mind is the master weaver, both of the inner garment of character and the outer garment of circumstance, and that, as they may have hitherto woven in ignorance and pain they may now weave in enlightenment and happiness.

JAMES ALLEN.

BROAD PARK AVENUE,

ILFRACOMBE, ENGLAND

AS A MAN THINKETH

THOUGHT AND CHARACTER

The aphorism, "As a man thinketh in his heart so is he," not only embraces the whole of a man's being, but is so comprehensive as to reach out to every condition and circumstance of his life. A man is literallywhat he thinks, his character being the complete sum of all his thoughts.

As the plant springs from, and could not be without, the seed, so every act of a man springs from the hidden seeds of thought, and could not have appeared without them. This applies equally to those acts called "spontaneous" and "unpremeditated" as to those, which are deliberately executed.

Act is the blossom of thought, and joy and suffering are its fruits; thus does a man garner in the sweet and bitter fruitage of his own husbandry.

"Thought in the mind hath made us, What we are by thought was wrought and built. If a man's mind hath evil thoughts, pain comes on him as comes the wheel the ox behind...if one endure in purity of thought, joy follows him as his own shadow sure."

Man is a growth by law, and not a creation by artifice, and cause and effect is as absolute and undeviating in the hidden realm of thought as in the world of visible and material things. A noble and Godlike character is not a thing of favour or chance, but is the natural result of continued effort in right thinking, the effect of long cherished association with Godlike thoughts. An ignoble and bestial character, by the same process, is the result of the continued harbouring of grovelling thoughts. Man is made or unmade by himself; in the armory of thought he forges the weapons by which he destroys himself; he also fashions the tools with which he builds for himself heavenly mansions of joy and strength and peace. By the right choice and true application of thought, man ascends to the Divine Perfection; by the abuse and wrong application of thought, he descends below the level of the beast. Between these two extremes are all the grades of character, and man is their maker and master.

Of all the beautiful truths pertaining to the soul which have been restored and brought to light in this age, none is more gladdening or fruitful of divine promise and confidence than this that man is the master of thought, the molder of character, and the maker and shaper of condition, environment, and destiny.

As a being of Power, Intelligence, and Love, and the lord of his own thoughts, man holds the key to every situation, and contains within himself that transforming and regenerative agency by which he may make himself what he wills.

Man is always the master, even in his weaker and most abandoned state; but in his weakness and degradation he is the foolish master who misgoverns his "household." When he begins to reflect upon his condition, and to search diligently for the Law upon which his being is established, he then becomes the wise master, directing his energies with intelligence, and fashioning his thoughts to fruitful issues. Such is the conscious master, and man can only thus become by discovering within himself the laws of thought; which discovery is totally a matter of application,self analysis, and experience.

Only by much searching and mining, are gold and diamonds obtained, and man can find everytruth connected with his being, if he will dig deep into the mine of his soul; and that he is the maker of his character, the moulder of his life, and the builder of his destiny, he may unerringly prove, if he will watch, control, and alter his thoughts, tracing their effects upon himself, upon others, and upon his life and circumstances, linking cause and effect by patient practice and investigation, and utilizing his every experience, even to the most trivial, everyday occurrence, as a means of obtaining that knowledge of himself which is Understanding, Wisdom, Power. In this direction, as in no other, is the law absolute that "He that seeketh findeth; and to him that knocketh it shall be opened;" for only by patience, practice, and ceaseless importunity can a man enter the Door of the Temple of Knowledge.

EFFECT OF THOUGHT ON CIRCUMSTANCES

MAN'S mind may be likened to a garden, which may be intelligently cultivated or allowed to run wild; but whether cultivated or neglected, it must, and will, bring forth.If no useful seeds are put into it, then an abundance of useless weed seeds will fall therein, and will continue to produce their kind. Just as a gardener cultivates his plot, keeping it free from weeds, and growing the flowers and fruits which he requires, so may a man tend the garden of his mind, weeding out all the wrong, useless, and impure thoughts, and cultivating toward perfection the flowers and fruits of right,useful, and pure thoughts. By pursuing this process, a man sooner or later discovers that he is the master gardener of his soul, the director of his life. He also reveals, within himself, the laws of thought, and understands, with ever increasing accuracy, how the thought forces and mind elements operate in the shaping of his character, circumstances, and destiny.

Thought and character are one, and as character can only manifest and discover itself through environment and circumstance, the outer conditions of a person's life will always be found to be harmoniously related to his inner state. This does not mean that a man's circumstances at any given time are an indication of his entire character, but that those circumstances are so intimately connected with some vital thought element within himself that, for the time being, they are indispensable to his development.

Every man is where he is by the law of his being; the thoughts which he has built into his character have brought him there, and in the arrangement of his life there is no element of chance, but all is the result of a law which cannot err. This is just as true of those who feel "out of harmony" with their surroundings as of those who are contented with them.

As a progressive and evolving being, man is where he is that he may learn that he may grow; and as he learns the spiritual lesson which any circumstance contains for him, it passes away and gives place to other circumstances.

Man is buffeted by circumstances so long as he believes himself to be the creature of outside conditions, but when he realizes that he is a creative power, and that he may command the hidden soil and seeds of his being out of which circumstances grow, he then becomes the rightful master of himself.

That circumstances grow out of thought every man knows who has for any length of time practiced self control and self purification, for he will have noticed that the alteration in his circumstances has been in exact ratio with his altered mental condition. So true is this that when a man earnestly applies himself to remedy the defects in his character, and makes swift and marked progress, he passes rapidly through a succession of vicissitudes.

The soul attracts that which it secretly harbours; that which it loves, and also that which it fears; it reaches the height of its cherished aspirations; it falls to the level of its unchastened desires, and circumstances are the means by which the soul receives its own.

Every thought seed sown or allowed to fall into the mind, and to take root there, produces its own, blossoming sooner or later into act, and bearing its own fruitage of opportunity and circumstance. Good thoughts bear good fruit, bad thoughts bad fruit.

The outer world of circumstance shapes itself to the inner world of thought, and both pleasant and unpleasant external conditions are factors, which make for the ultimate good of the individual. As the reaper of his own harvest, man learns both by suffering and bliss.

Following the inmost desires, aspirations, thoughts, by which he allows himself to be dominated, (pursuing the will o' the wisps of impure imaginings or steadfastly walking the highway of strong and high endeavour), a man at last arrives at their fruition and fulfilment in the outerconditions of his life. The laws of growth and adjustment everywhere obtains.

A man does not come to the almshouse or the jail by the tyranny of fate or circumstance, but by the pathway of grovelling thoughts and base desires. Nor does a pure minded man fall suddenly into crime by stress of any mere external force; the criminal thought had long been secretly fostered in the heart, and the hour of opportunity revealed its gathered power. Circumstance does not make the man; it reveals him to himself No such conditions can exist as descending into vice and its attendant sufferings apart from vicious inclinations, or ascending into virtue and its pure happiness without the continued cultivation of virtuous aspirations; and man, therefore, as the lord and master of thought, is the maker of himself the shaper and author of environment. Even at birth the soul comes to its own and through every step of its earthly pilgrimage it attracts those combinations of conditions which reveal itself, which are the reflections of its own purity and, impurity, its strength and weakness. Men do not attract that which theywant, but that which they are.

Their whims, fancies, and ambitions are thwarted at every step, but their inmost thoughts and desires are fed with their own food, be it foul or clean. The "divinity that shapes our ends" is in ourselves; it is our very self.

Only himself manacles man: thought and action are the gaolers of Fate they imprison, being base; they are also the angels of Freedom they liberate, being noble. Not what he wishes and prays for does a man get, but what he justly earns. His wishes and prayers are only gratified and answered when they harmonize with his thoughts and actions.

In the light of this truth, what, then, is the meaning of "fighting against circumstances?" It means that a man is continually revolting against an effect without, while all the time he is nourishing and preserving its cause in his heart. That cause may take the form of a conscious vice or an unconscious weakness; but whatever it is, it stubbornly retards the efforts of its possessor, and thus calls aloud for remedy.

Men are anxious to improve their circumstances, but are unwilling to improve themselves; they therefore remain bound. The man who does not shrink from self-crucifixion can never fail to accomplish the object upon which his heart is set. This is as true of earthly as of heavenly things.

Even the man whose sole object is to acquire wealth must be prepared to make great personal sacrifices before he can accomplish his object; and how much more so he who would realize a strong and well poised life?

Here is a man who is wretchedly poor. He is extremely anxious that his surroundings and home comforts should be improved, yet all the time he shirks his work, and considers he is justified in trying to deceive his employer on the ground of the insufficiency of his wages. Such a man does not understand the simplest rudiments of those principles which are the basis of true prosperity, and is not only totally unfitted to rise out of his wretchedness, but is actually attracting to himself a still deeper wretchedness by dwelling in, and acting out, indolent, deceptive, and unmanly thoughts.

Here is a rich man who is the victim of a painful and persistent disease as the result of gluttony. He is willing to give large sums of money to get rid of it, but he will not sacrifice his gluttonous desires. He wants to gratify his taste for rich and unnatural viands and have his health as well. Such a man is totally unfit to have health, because he has not yet learned the first principles of a healthy life.

Here is an employer of labour who adopts crooked measures to avoid paying the regulation wage, and, in the hope of making larger profits, reduces the wages of his workpeople. Such a man is altogether unfitted for prosperity, and when he finds himself bankrupt, both as regards reputation and riches, he blames circumstances, not knowing that he is the sole author of his condition.

I have introduced these three cases merely as illustrative of the truth that man is the causer (though nearly always is unconsciously) of his circumstances, and that, whilst aiming at a goodend, he is continually frustrating its accomplishment by encouraging thoughts and desires which cannot possibly harmonize with that end. Such cases could be multiplied and varied almost indefinitely, but this is not necessary, as the reader can, if he so resolves, trace the action of the laws of thought in his own mind and life, and until this is done, mere external facts cannot serve as a ground of reasoning.

Circumstances, however, are so complicated, thought is so deeply rooted, and the conditions of happiness vary so, vastly with individuals, that a man's entire soul condition (although it may be known to himself) cannot be judged by another from the external aspect of his life alone. A man may be honest in certain directions, yet suffer privations; a man may be dishonest in certain directions, yet acquire wealth; but the conclusion usually formed that the one man fails because of his particular honesty, and that the other prospers because of his particular dishonesty, is the result of a superficial judgment, which assumes that the dishonest man is almost totally corrupt, and the honest man almost entirely virtuous. In the light of a deeper knowledge and wider experience such judgment is found to be erroneous. The dishonest man may have some admirable virtues, which the other does, not possess; and the honest man obnoxious vices which are absent in the other. The honest man reaps the good results of his honest thoughts and acts; he also brings upon himself the sufferings, which his vices produce. The dishonest man likewise garners his own suffering and happiness.

It is pleasing to human vanity to believe that one suffers because of one's virtue; but not until a man has extirpated every sickly, bitter, and impure thought from his mind, and washed every sinful stain from his soul, can he be in a position to know and declare that his sufferings are the result of his good, and not of his bad qualities; and on the way to, yet long before he has reached, that supreme perfection, he will have found, working in his mind and life, the Great Law which is absolutely just, and which cannot, therefore, give good for evil, evil for good. Possessed of

such knowledge, he will then know, looking back upon his past ignorance and blindness, that his life is, and always was, justly ordered, and that all his past experiences, good and bad, were the equitable outworking of his evolving, yet unevolved self. Good thoughts and actions can never produce bad results; bad thoughts and actions can never produce good results. This is but saying that nothing can come from corn but corn, nothing from nettles but nettles. Men understand this law in the natural world, and work with it; but few understand it in the mental and moral world (though its operation there is just as simple and undeviating), and they, therefore, do not cooperate with it.

Suffering is always the effect of wrong thought in some direction. It is an indication that the individual is out of harmony with himself, with the Law of his being. The sole and supreme use of suffering is to purify, to burn out all that is useless and impure. Suffering ceases for him who is pure. There could be no object in burning gold after the dross had been removed, and a perfectly pure and enlightened being could not suffer.

The circumstances, which a man encounters with suffering, are the result of his own mental in harmony. The circumstances, which a man encounters with blessedness, are the result of his own mental harmony. Blessedness, not material possessions, is the measure of right thought; wretchedness, not lack of material possessions, is the measure of wrong thought. A man may be cursed and rich; he may be blessed and poor. Blessedness and riches are only joined together when the riches are rightly and wisely used; and the poor man only descends into wretchedness when he regards his lot as a burden unjustly imposed.

Indigence and indulgence are the two extremes of wretchedness. They are both equally unnatural and the result of mental disorder. A man is not rightly conditioned until he is a happy, healthy, and prosperous being; and happiness, health, and prosperity are the result of a harmonious adjustment of the inner with the outer, of the man with his surroundings.

A man only begins to be a man when he ceases to whine and revile, and commences to search for the hidden justice which regulates his life. And as he adapts his mind to that regulating factor, he ceases to accuse others as the cause of his condition, and builds himself up in strong and noble thoughts; ceases to kick against circumstances, but begins to use them as aids to his more rapid progress, and as a means of discovering the hidden powers and possibilities within himself.

Law, not confusion, is the dominating principle in the universe; justice, not injustice, is the soul and substance of life; and righteousness, not corruption, is the moulding and moving force in the spiritual government of the world. This being so, man has but to right himself to find that the universe is right; and during the process of putting himself right he will find that as he alters his thoughts towards things and other people, things and other people will alter towards him.

The proof of this truth is in every person, and it therefore admits of easy investigation by systematic introspection and self analysis. Let a man radically alter his thoughts, and he will be astonished at the rapid transformation it will effect in the material conditions of his life. Men imagine that thought can be kept secret, but it cannot; it rapidly crystallizes into habit, and habit solidifies into circumstance. Bestial thoughts crystallize into habits of drunkenness and sensuality, which solidify into circumstances of destitution and disease: impure thoughts of every kind crystallize into enervating and confusing habits, which solidify into distracting and adverse circumstances: thoughts of fear, doubt, and indecision crystallize into weak, unmanly, and irresolute habits, which solidify into circumstances of failure, indigence, and slavish dependence: lazy thoughts crystallize into habits of uncleanliness and dishonesty, which solidify into circumstances of foulness and beggary: hateful and condemnatory thoughts crystallize in to habits of accusation and violence, which solidify into circumstances of injury and persecution: selfish thoughts of all kinds crystallize into habits of self seeking, which solidify into circumstances more or less distressing. On the other hand, beautiful thoughts of all kinds crystallize into habits of grace and kindliness, which solidify into genial and sunny circumstances: pure thoughts crystallize into habits of temperance and selfcontrol, which solidify into circumstances of repose and peace: thoughts of courage, self reliance, and decision crystallize into manly habits, which solidify into circumstances of success, plenty, and freedom: energetic thoughts crystallize into habits of cleanliness and industry, which solidify into circumstances of pleasantness: gentle and forgiving thoughts crystallize into habits of gentleness, which solidify into protective and preservative circumstances: loving and unselfish thoughts crystallize into habits of self forgetfulness for others, which solidify into circumstances of sure and abiding prosperity and true riches.

A particular train of thought persisted in, be it good or bad, cannot fail to produce its results on the character and circumstances. A man cannot directly choose his circumstances, but he can choose his thoughts, and so indirectly, yet surely, shape his circumstances.

Nature helps every man to the gratification of the thoughts, which he most encourages, and opportunities are presented which will most speedily bring to the surface both the good and evil thoughts.

Let a man cease from his sinful thoughts, and all the world will soften towards him, and be ready to help him; let him put away his weakly and sickly thoughts, and lo, opportunities will spring up on every hand to aid his strong resolves; let him encourage good thoughts, and no hard fate shall bind him down to wretchedness and shame. The world is your kaleidoscope, and the varying combinations of colours, which at every succeeding moment it presents to you are the exquisitely adjusted pictures of your ever moving thoughts.

> "So You will be what you will to be;
> Let failure find its false content

In that poor word, 'environment,'
But spirit scorns it, and is free.
"It masters time, it conquers space;
It cowes that boastful trickster, Chance,
And bids the tyrant Circumstance
Uncrown, and fill a servant's place.
"The human Will, that force unseen,
The offspring of a deathless Soul,
Can hew a way to any goal,
Though walls of granite intervene.
"Be not impatient in delays
But wait as one who understands;
When spirit rises and commands
The gods are ready to obey."

EFFECT OF THOUGHT ON HEALTH AND THE BODY

THE body is the servant of the mind. It obeys the operations of the mind, whether they be deliberately chosen or automatically expressed. At the bidding of unlawful thoughts the body sinks rapidly into disease and decay; at the command of glad and beautiful thoughts it becomes clothed with youthfulness and beauty.

Disease and health, like circumstances, are rooted in thought. Sickly thoughts will express themselves through a sickly body. Thoughts of fear have been known to kill a man as speedily as a bullet, and they are continually killing thousands of people just as surely though less rapidly.

The people who live in fear of disease are the people who get it. Anxiety quickly demoralizes the whole body, and lays it open to the entrance of disease; while impure thoughts, even if not physically indulged, will soon shatter the nervous system.

Strong, pure, and happy thoughts build up the body in vigour and grace. The body is a delicate and plastic instrument, which responds readily to the thoughts by which it is impressed, and habits of thought will produce their own effects, good or bad, upon it.

Men will continue to have impure and poisoned blood, so long as they propagate unclean thoughts. Out of a clean heart comes a clean life and a clean body. Out of a defiled mind proceeds a defiled life and a corrupt body. Thought is the fount of action, life, and manifestation; make the fountain pure, and all will be pure.

Change of diet will not help a man who will not change his thoughts. When a man makes his thoughts pure, he no longer desires impure food.

Clean thoughts make clean habits. The so called saint who does not wash his body is not a saint.

He who has strengthened and purified his thoughts does not need to consider the malevolent microbe.

If you would protect your body, guard your mind. If you would renew your body, beautify your mind. Thoughts of malice, envy, disappointment, despondency, rob the body of its health and grace. A sour face does not come by chance; it is made by sour thoughts. Wrinkles that mar are drawn by folly, passion, and pride.

I know a woman of ninety six who has the bright, innocent face of a girl. I know a man well under middle age whose face is drawn into inharmonious contours. The one is the result of a sweet and sunny disposition; the other is the outcome of passion and discontent.

As you cannot have a sweet and wholesome abode unless you admit the air and sunshine freely into your rooms, so a strong body and a bright, happy, or serene countenance can only result from the free admittance into the mind of thoughts of joy and goodwill and serenity.

On the faces of the aged there are wrinkles made by sympathy, others by strong and pure thought, and others are carved by passion: who cannot distinguish them? With those who have lived righteously, age is calm, peaceful, and softly mellowed, like the setting sun. I have recently seen a philosopher on his deathbed. He was not old except in years. He died as sweetly and peacefully as he had lived.

There is no physician like cheerful thought for dissipating the ills of the body; there is no comforter to compare with goodwill for dispersing the shadows of grief and sorrow. To live continually in thoughts of ill will, cynicism, suspicion, and envy, is to be confined in a self made prison hole. But to think well of all, to be cheerful with all, to patiently learn to find the good in all such unselfish thoughts are the very portals of heaven; and to dwell day by day in thoughts of peace toward every creature will bring abounding peace to their possessor.

THOUGHT AND PURPOSE

UNTIL thought is linked with purpose there is no intelligent accomplishment. With the majority the bark of thought is allowed to "drift" upon the ocean of life. Aimlessness is a vice, and such drifting must not continue for him who would steer clear of catastrophe and destruction.

They who have no central purpose in their life fall an easy prey to petty worries, fears, troubles, and self pityings, all of which are indications of weakness, which lead, just as surely as deliberately planned sins (though by a different route), to failure, unhappiness, and loss, for weakness cannot persist in a power evolving universe.

A man should conceive of a legitimate purpose in his heart, and set out to accomplish it. He should make this purpose the centralizing point of his thoughts. It may take the form of a spiritual ideal, or it may be a worldly object, according to his nature at the time being; but whichever it is, he should steadily focus his thought forces upon the object, which he has set before him. He should make this purpose his supreme duty, and should devote himself to its attainment, not allowing his thoughts to wander away into ephemeral fancies, longings, and imaginings. This is the royal road to self control and true concentration of thought. Even if he fails again and again to accomplish his purpose (as he necessarily must until weakness is overcome), the strength of character gained will be the measure of his true success, and this will form a new starting point for future power and triumph. Those who are not prepared for the apprehension of a great purpose should fix the thoughts upon the faultless performance of their duty, no matter how insignificant their task may appear. Only in this way can the thoughts be gathered and focused, and resolution and energy be developed, which being done, there is nothing which may not be accomplished.

The weakest soul, knowing its own weakness, and believing this truth that strength can only be developed by effort and practice, will, thus believing, at once begin to exert itself, and, adding effort to effort, patience to patience, and strength to strength, will never cease to develop, and will at last grow divinely strong.

As the physically weak man can make himself strong by careful and patient training, so the man of weak thoughts can make them strong by exercising himself in right thinking.

To put away aimlessness and weakness, and to begin to think with purpose, is to enter the ranks of those strong ones who only recognize failure as one of the pathways to attainment; who make all conditions serve them, and who think strongly, attempt fearlessly, and accomplish masterfully.

Having conceived of his purpose, a man should mentally mark out a straight pathway to its achievement, looking neither to the right nor the left. Doubts and fear s should be rigorously excluded; they are disintegrating elements, which break up the straight line of effort, rendering it crooked, ineffectual, useless. Thoughts of doubt and fear never accomplished anything, and never can. They always lead to failure. Purpose, energy, power to do, and all strong thoughts cease when doubt and fear creep in.

The will to do springs from the knowledge that we can do. Doubt and fear are the great enemies of knowledge, and he who encourages them, who does not slay them, thwarts himself at every step.

He who has conquered doubt and fear has conquered failure. His every thought is allied with power, and all difficulties are bravely met and wisely overcome. His purposes are seasonably planted, and they bloom and bring forth fruit, which does not fall prematurely to the ground.

Thought allied fearlessly to purpose becomes creative force: he who knows this is ready to become something higher and stronger than a mere bundle of wavering thoughts and fluctuating sensations; he who does this has become the conscious and intelligent wielder of his mental powers.

THE THOUGHT: FACTOR IN ACHIEVEMENT

ALL that a man achieves and all that he fails to achieve is the direct result of his own thoughts. In a justly ordered universe, where loss of equipoise would mean total destruction, individual

responsibility must be absolute. A man's weakness and strength, purity and impurity, are his own, and not another man's; they are brought about by himself, and not by another; and they can only be altered by himself, never by another. His condition is also his own, and not another man's. His suffering and his happiness are evolved from within. As he thinks, so he is; as he continues to think, so he remains.

A strong man cannot help a weaker unless that weaker is willing to be helped, and even then the weak man must become strong of himself; he must, by his own efforts, develop the strength which he admires in another. None but himself can alter his condition.

It has been usual for men to think and to say, "Many men are slaves because one is an oppressor; let us hate the oppressor." Now, however, there is amongst an increasing few a tendency to reverse this judgment, and to say, "One man is an oppressor because many are slaves; let us despise the slaves."

The truth is that oppressor and slave are cooperators in ignorance, and, while seeming to afflict each other, are in reality afflicting themselves. A perfect Knowledge perceives the action of law in the weakness of the oppressed and the misapplied power of the oppressor; a perfect Love, seeing the suffering, which both states entail, condemns neither; a perfect Compassion embraces both oppressor and oppressed.

He who has conquered weakness, and has put away all selfish thoughts, belongs neither tooppressor nor oppressed. He is free.

A man can only rise, conquer, and achieve by lifting up his thoughts. He can only remain weak, and abject, and miserable by refusing to lift up his thoughts.

Before a man can achieve anything, even in worldly things, he must lift his thoughts above slavish animal indulgence. He may not, in order to succeed, give up all animality and selfishness, by any means; but a portion of it must, at least, be sacrificed. A man whose first thought is bestial indulgence could neither think clearly nor plan methodically; he could not find and develop his latent resources, and would fail in any undertaking. Not having commenced to manfully control his thoughts, he is not in a position to control affairs and to adopt serious responsibilities. He is not fit to act independently and stand alone. But he is limited only by the thoughts, which he chooses.

There can be no progress, no achievement without sacrifice, and a man's worldly success will be in the measure that he sacrifices his confused animal thoughts, and fixes his mind on the development of his plans, and the strengthening of his resolution and self reliance. And the higher he lifts his thoughts, the more manly, upright, and righteous he becomes, the greater will be his success, the more blessed and enduring will be his achievements.

The universe does not favour the greedy, the dishonest, the vicious, although on the mere surface it may sometimes appear to do so; it helps the honest, the magnanimous, the virtuous. All the great Teachers of the ages have declared this in varying forms, and to prove and know it a manhas but to persist in making himself more and more virtuous by lifting up his thoughts.

Intellectual achievements are the result of thought consecrated to the search for knowledge, or for the beautiful and true in life and nature. Such achievements may be sometimes connected with vanity and ambition, but they are not the outcome of those characteristics; they are thenatural outgrowth of long and arduous effort, and of pure and unselfish thoughts.

Spiritual achievements are the consummation of holy aspirations. He who lives constantly in the conception of noble and lofty thoughts, who dwells upon all that is pure and unselfish, will, as surely as the sun reaches its zenith and the moon its full, become wise and noble in character, and rise into a position of influence and blessedness.

Achievement, of whatever kind, is the crown of effort, the diadem of thought. By the aid of self control, resolution, purity, righteousness, and well directed thought a man ascends; by the aid ofanimality, indolence, impurity, corruption, and confusion of thought a man descends.

A man may rise to high success in the world, and even to lofty altitudes in the spiritual realm, and again descend into weakness and wretchedness by allowing arrogant, selfish, and corrupt thoughts to take possession of him.

Victories attained by right thought can only be maintained by watchfulness. Many give waywhen success is assured, and rapidly fall back into failure.

All achievements, whether in the business, intellectual, or spiritual world, are the result of definitely directed thought, are governed by the same law and are of the same method; the only difference lies in the object of attainment.

He who would accomplish little must sacrifice little; he who would achieve much must sacrifice much; he who would attain highly must sacrifice greatly.

VISIONS AND IDEALS

THE dreamers are the saviours of the world. As the visible world is sustained by the invisible, so men, through all their trials and sins and sordid vocations, are nourished by the beautiful visions of their solitary dreamers. Humanity cannot forget its dreamers; it cannot let their ideals fade and die; it lives in them; it knows them as they realities which it shall one day see and know.

Composer, sculptor, painter, poet, prophet, sage, these are the makers ofthe after world, the architects of heaven. The world is beautiful because they have lived; without them, labouring humanity would perish.

He who cherishes a beautiful vision, a lofty ideal in his heart, will one day realize it. Columbus cherished a vision of another world, and he discovered it; Copernicus fostered the vision of a multiplicity of worlds and a wider universe, and he revealed it; Buddha beheld the vision of a spiritual world of stainless beauty and perfect peace, and he entered into it.

Cherish your visions; cherish your ideals; cherish the music that stirs in your heart, the beauty that forms in your mind, the loveliness that drapes your purest thoughts, for out of them will grow all delightful conditions, all, heavenly environment; of these, if you but remain true to them, your world will at last be built.

To desire is to obtain; to aspire is to, achieve. Shall man's basest desires receive the fullest measure of gratification, and his purest aspirations starve for lack of sustenance? Such is not the Law: such a condition of things can never obtain: "ask and receive."

Dream lofty dreams, and as you dream, so shall you become Your Vision is the promise of what you shall one day be; your Ideal is the prophecy of what you shall at last unveil. The greatest achievement was at first and for a time a dream. The oak sleeps in the acorn; thebird waits in the egg; and in the highest vision of the soul a waking angel stirs. Dreams are the seedlings of realities.

Your circumstances may be uncongenial, but they shall not long remain so if you but perceive an Ideal and strive to reach it. You cannot travel within and stand still without.

Here is a youth hard pressed by poverty and labour; confined long hours in an unhealthy workshop; unschooled, and lacking all the arts of refinement. But he dreams of better things; he thinks of intelligence, of refinement, of grace and beauty. He conceives of, mentally builds up, an ideal condition of life; the vision of a wider liberty and a larger scope takes possession of him; unrest urges him to action, and he utilizes all his spare time and means, small though they are, to the development of his latent powers and resources. Very soon so altered has his mind become that the workshop can no longer hold him. It has become so out of harmony with his mentality that it falls out of his life as a garment is cast aside, and, with the growth of opportunities, which fit the scope of his expanding powers, he passes out of it forever. Years later we see this youth as a full grown man.

We find him a master of certain forces of the mind, which he wields with worldwide influence and almost unequalled power. In his hands he holds the cords of gigantic responsibilities; he speaks, and lo, lives are changed;

men and women hang upon his words and remould their characters, and, sunlike, he becomes the fixed and luminous centre round which innumerable destinies revolve. He has realized the Vision of his youth. He has become one with his Ideal. And you, too, youthful reader, will realize the Vision (not the idle wish) of your heart, be it base or beautiful, or a mixture of both, for you will always gravitate toward that which you, secretly, most love. Into your hands will be placed the exact results of your own thoughts; you will receive that which you earn; no more, no less. Whatever your present environment may be, you will fall, remain, or rise with your thoughts, your Vision, your Ideal. You will become as small as your controlling desire; as great as your dominant aspiration: in the beautiful words of Stanton Kirkham Davis, "You may be keeping accounts, and presently you shall walk out of the door that for so long has seemed to you the barrier of your ideals, and shall find yourself before an audience the pen still behind your ear, the ink stains on your fingers and then and there shall pour out the torrent of your inspiration. You may be driving sheep, and you shall wander to the city bucolic and open-mouthed; shall wander under the intrepid guidance of the spirit into the studio of the master, and after a time he shall say, 'I have nothing more to teach you.' And now you have become the master, who did so recently dream of great things while driving sheep. You shall lay down the saw and the plane to take upon yourself the regeneration of the world."

The thoughtless, the ignorant, and the indolent, seeing only the apparent effects of things and not the things themselves, talk of luck, of fortune, and chance. Seeing a man grow rich, they say, "How lucky he is!" Observing another become intellectual, they exclaim, "How highly favoured he is!" And noting the saintly character and wide influence of another, they remark, "How chance aids him at every turn!" They do not see the trials and failures and struggles which these men have voluntarily encountered in order to gain their experience; have no knowledge of the sacrifices they have made, of the undaunted efforts they have put forth, of the faith they have exercised, that they might overcome the apparently insurmountable, and realize the Vision of their heart. They do not know the darkness and the heartaches; they only see the light and joy, and call it "luck". They do not see the long and arduous journey, but only behold the pleasant goal, and call it "good fortune," do not understand the process, but only perceive the result, and call it chance. In all human affairs there are efforts, and there are results, and the strength of the effort is the measure of the result. Chance is not. Gifts, powers, material, intellectual, and spiritual possessions are the fruits of effort; they are thoughts completed, objects accomplished, visions realized.

The Vision that you glorify in your mind, the Ideal that you enthrone in your heart this you will build your life by, this you will become. SERENITY CALMNESS of mind is one of the beautiful jewels of wisdom. It is the result of long and patient effort in selfcontrol. Its presence is an indication of ripened experience, and of a more than ordinary knowledge of the laws and operations of thought. A man becomes calm in the measure that he understands himself as a thought evolved being, for such knowledge necessitates the understanding of others as the result of thought, and as he develops a right understanding, and sees more and more clearly the internal relations of things by the action of cause and effect he ceases to fuss and fume and worry and grieve, and remains poised, steadfast, serene.

The calm man, having learned how to govern himself, knows how to adapt himself to others; and they, in turn, reverence his spiritual strength, and feel that they can learn of him and rely upon him. The more tranquil a man becomes, the greater is his success, his influence, his power for good. Even the ordinary trader will find his business prosperity increase as he develops a greaterself control and equanimity, for people will always prefer to deal with a man whose demeanour is strongly equable.

Inner Game of Weight Loss Wrestling Agreement

CoCreated with You & Your Coach

The following agreement made on _____ of_____ 2015 between Brian Daly, _____ (Student Athlete) and_____. (Parent)

Parent Signature _____

Student Signature _____

Application Approval Signature _____

Intention:

To Develop You the Leader Within You

Outcomes:

1. You will experience a positive winning culture that causes you to stretch your vision of what's possible.

2. You will know yourself as a leader, with an increase in confidence and the ability to trust your training in the moments that matter most.

3. You will breakthrough any limiting beliefs that are holding you back.

☐ Yes Brian, I am choosing to do something different this year .

I am NOW making a 6 month commitment to you, my team, and myself. I am deciding to follow your process and I am coachable.

Student Athlete: _____

Parents Name: _____

Address:_____

City: _____ State: _____ Zip:_____

E-mail*: _____

Phone: _____

Credit Card: (check one)
Visa: _____   MasterCard: _____ Other: _____

3 Digit Code: _____

Amount Today $_____

Credit Card Number: _____

Exp. Date: _____

Signature: _____

Date: _____

*Providing this information constitutes your permission for The Inner Game of Weight Loss contact you regarding related information via mail, e-mail, fax, and phone

About The Author:

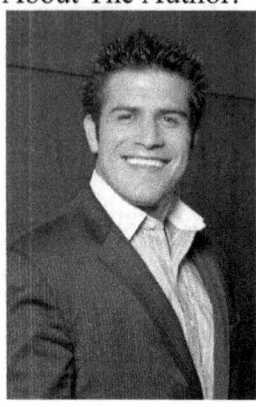

Brian Daly Entrepreneur, Author & Founder & Lead Coach for The Inner Game of Weight Loss™.

For close to a decade, Brian competed as a top Nationally-Ranked Wrestler, where he competed 4x's at the NCAA National Championships, was invited 2x's to the largest Division I NCAA Championship Tournament, and received the U.S. Marine Corp Award.

These may seem like great accomplishments for any individual, however Brian saw it differently. Each and every year for 7 years straight, he qualified for the High School State and College NCAA National Championships. And each and every year, Brian was unable to achieve his goal of being an All-American or National Champion. When it came down to the most critical moments of competition, there was always something that just seemed to happen, leaving Brian disappointed and with many unanswered questions.

Brian's purpose in life is to work with wrestlers and develop their leadership, a positive mental attitude & expose them to the possibilities of being an Entrepreneur. He believes being an entrepreneur is the solution to the challenges with the current educations system.

Brian a Coach, Entrepreneur & Author of 2 Books, **"The Inner Game of Weight Loss™"** & Forth coming book **"3 Day MBA"** Everything You Will Never Get From Business School www.3DayMBABook.com

Brian currently lives in Chicago, IL near Midway Airport and married to his beautiful wife Francielle, has two girls, 6 year old daughter Nelyssa and new born baby girl Genesis.

The Inner Game of Weight Loss™

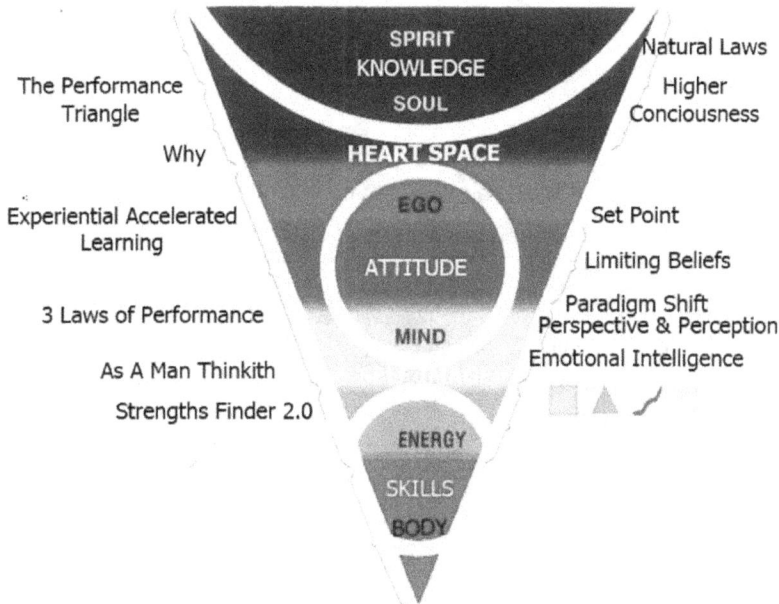

"Now Claim Your Free Strategy Session to Experience the Power of Your Personality & See For the 1ˢᵗ Time Ever Your Preferred Coaching Style"

Many times this call looks like a 30 minute call between you and our leadership team.

To Schedule a time that works for everyone
Call 773-574-6600.

" Or To Apply to The Inner Game of Weight Loss™ Team"

Visit: